DR. KNOWWHY

So You Think You Want to Be a Doctor?

13 Reasons You Might Want to Reconsider

This book was professionally typeset on Reedsy.
Find out more at reedsy.com

Contents

1

Introduction

The Fantasy

Once upon a time, I wanted to be a medical doctor. I wanted it BIG TIME. But I knew the competition to get into medical school was insane, so I didn't go around telling people it was my dream. That way, if I didn't make it, no one would know what a failure I was.

But during the summer after I graduated from college, I went home for lunch one day and found a telegram stuck on my door. It was from a medical school, and it said: "HAS INSTRUCTED ME TO ADVISE YOU THAT YOU ARE HEREBY OFFERED A POSITION IN THE FRESHMAN CLASS OF 1972-73…" I know what it said because I still have the telegram. What I don't know is - what's the subject of that sentence? Who instructed the writer to make the offer? I guess I'll never know.

I wasn't over the moon - I was over *Jupiter*! I had been accepted into medical school! I was so thrilled, excited, and agog with joy that I actually wrote this bit of doggerel to commemorate the occasion:

When Dreams Come True

You will dream it for a lifetime -
   You will hope, and wish, and pray.
   Then suddenly it is before you -
   A letter, a telegram, a message will say:

"Awake, dreamer of beautiful dreams. Awake!
   The dream is over, life to begin.
   The world is made of rainbows today -
   Beckoning, but scattered before the wind.

"Awake. Your one, great dream is fulfilled today,
   And there is a beautiful work to do.
   Put all other dreams aside
   And prepare for the task God has chosen for you."

Then your heart will sing like the nightingale,
   You will dance as the wild winds blow,
   You will look to Heaven and whisper,
   "Someone does care, and now I know!"

The Reality

At the age of 70-something, I'm grateful every day I wake up and still remember who I am. Yet I have a crystal clear memory of two things from my first day in medical school, 50+ years ago.

The first thing I remember is this statement: "I hope you got a good night's sleep last night because it's the last one you're going to get for the rest of your life." Gulp! I'd had a HORRIBLE night's sleep, as my restless mind was trying to prepare itself for my safari into the deep, dark Unknown.

The second thing I remember from that day was a discussion of cadavers. The anatomy professor was very stern - he did not want to EVER walk into the anatomy lab and find us throwing pancreases around. What a ridiculous thought! But my mind by-passed the gruesome image of flying body parts. It had frozen on the word "cadaver." Yikes! I was going to have to dissect a dead person!

"WHAT AM I DOING HERE?" was my silent scream.

I never found a good answer to that pounding question.

What WAS I Doing There?

My reasons for "being there" were probably typical of every other medical student in the room. First, we all cared very much about helping people. Disease and infirmity are monsters. Who wouldn't want to slay those dragons?

Then there was the perception of respect. 50 years ago, members of the medical profession were generally respected and looked up to. I was the teeniest, tiniest kind of Nobody. Becoming a doctor would surely turn me into a Somebody. Not much of a Somebody, of course, but at least, I wouldn't be a complete Nobody any more.

I still remember that once, back in my high school days, I suggested the possibility of becoming a nurse. A friend contradicted me immediately, "Oh no!" she exclaimed. "You're too smart to be a nurse. You should be a doctor!"

The explosion of ego edema was instantaneous. And foolish. There are plenty of nurses who are just as smart as doctors. Smarter - they were smart enough not to become doctors! And I will be forever indebted to the nurses who helped me survive my residency.

Anyway, for better or worse, I was there. And, as bad as the first day was, things only rolled downhill from that point.

13 Reasons You Might Not Want to Be a Doctor

Not all the reasons listed below affected me personally. I will certainly mention the things that impacted my life and thoughts. But people are so different it's only reasonable to throw in considerations that were not a problem for me, but might be a problem for others.

My list isn't exhaustive, but hopefully, it will alert you to a few issues you'll want to know about and consider before you find yourself face-to-face with a cadaver of your own.

Oh, and BTW, I finally decided there's only one good reason to become a practicing physician. I'll share that conclusion with you at the end of this book.

2

Reason #1 - Health? What's that?

I'll start with my number one complaint about being a doctor. Doctors don't know *anything* about health. Physicians are called doctors of medicine because they study medicine - diseases and the medicines used to treat diseases. Not once in my entire medical training did I hear a lecture on being healthy. On taking a non-diseased person and helping them be a healthier person. Or any related topic.

I had been out of medical school for several years before I put these puzzle pieces together. They weren't *supposed* to teach me about health, I finally realized. It was MEDICAL school.

But I wasn't interested in disease. I wasn't interested in drugs or surgery. I was interested in HEALTH.

My last year in medical school I went to the library several times and thumbed through numerous books, trying to find a specialty that appealed to me. It didn't exist. And I didn't realize why at the time.

A few years later, it began to dawn on me that if I was interested in health, I should be studying nutrition or fitness. I'm not particularly athletic, so I actually considered going back to school and taking a course in nutrition. But I had two problems with that idea:

One, I'd been in school 20 years, and it hadn't done me any good. So why should I think more school was a solution?

Two, every time you listened to the news, you heard contradictory nutritional reports. "Coffee is bad for you." "Coffee is good for you." "Eggs are bad for you." "Eggs are good for you." I wasn't convinced a nutrition education could be trusted. So I didn't bother.

BTW, In case you're interested, I've read some nutrition books in recent years, and I found out why there are so many contradictory "findings" in the area of nutrition. It seems that the big food producers are the ones who fund many of the "scientific" studies on foods, and those studies tend to magically support the foods produced by the companies paying the bills. Imagine that!

Here's something else I found out. If you don't eat anything that comes in bags or boxes, your health will probably benefit.

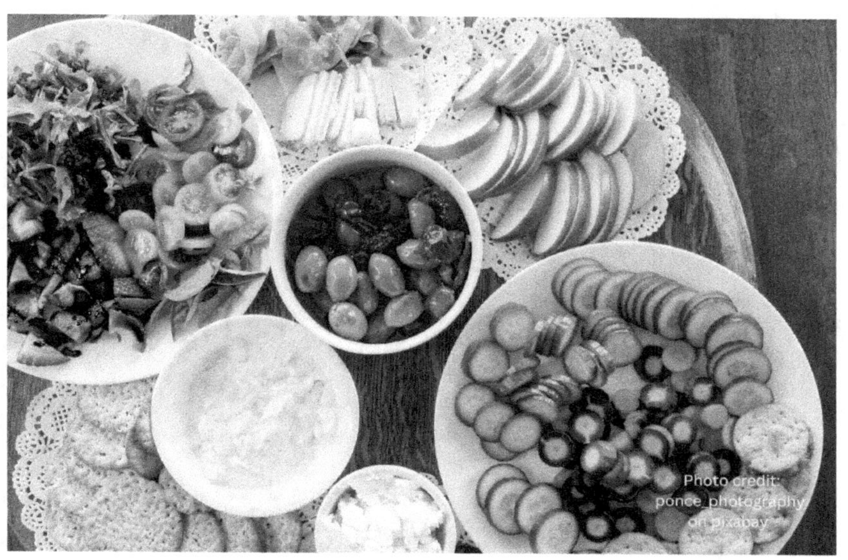
Photo credit:
ponce_photography
on pixabay

3

Reason # 2 - A Numbers' Game

Medicine is a number's game. That fact doesn't bother me because I like math, but it does amuse me. Nobody ever tells you how much medicine is about juggling numbers.

For example, say a child comes in with a temperature of 102 degrees. That's a number. The child's heart is beating at a rate of 100 beats per minute. That's a number. The child's respiration rate is 40 per minute. Another number.

So the doctor examines the child and decides she needs an antibiotic. He takes the child's weight - a number - and calculates the appropriate dosage in grams or milligrams - a number. He writes a prescription saying how many milliliters - a number - the child should swallow every 4 hours or every 6 hours - more numbers.

Or suppose an adult comes in and their blood pressure is too high - that's two numbers. The doctor prescribes a medication of a certain dosage - that's a number - and tells the patient the *number* of times per day to take it.

Lab tests are whole lists of numbers. The doctor looks at them: red blood count, white blood count, cholesterol level, hormone levels, etc. Numbers, numbers, numbers. And if a prescription is called for, how much is appropriate and how many times a day should the patient take it? More numbers.

Well, you get the idea. There really is a lot more to medicine than numbers, but if you don't like math, *Watch Out*!

4

Reason # 3 - The Hard Part

Do you remember how I said getting into medical school was so competitive I didn't even want anybody to know I was trying since I would probably fail? Well, it turns out that getting in was the easy part. The great powers-that-be who ordained it should be *hard, hard, hard* to get into their hallowed halls knew what they were doing. The hard part begins after you're in.

The first term of the first year consisted of lectures and labs. Three courses were dense, intense science courses - anatomy, biochemistry, and microbiology. In my entire educational career, I had made only a few grades below an A. For that term, I netted three C's, one B, an S, and a CR.

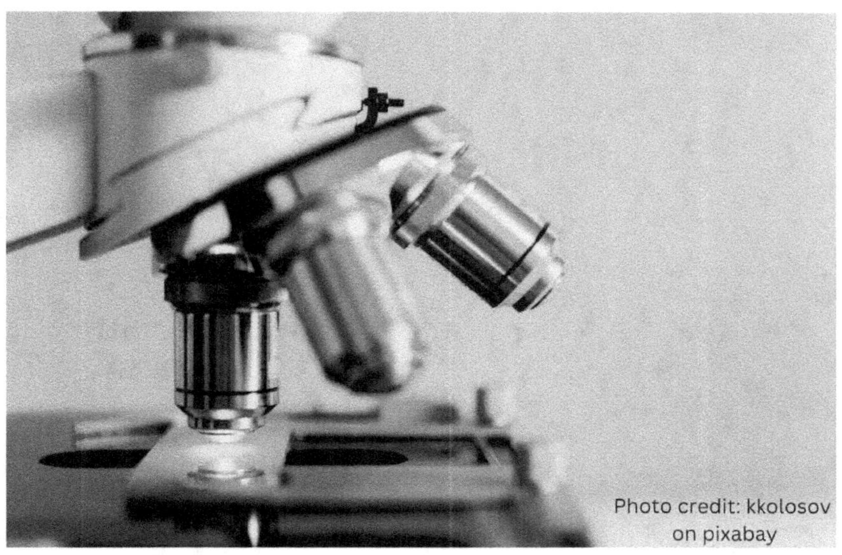

Photo credit: kkolosov
on pixabay

I was not a happy camper. But the next term was worse. I not only didn't make a single A, I failed physiology. Gasp! I had never imagined that I might be capable of *failing* a course. But I bombed physiology and had to take it again. Gloom, doom, and despair...

Okay, I was passing overall, but it was TOUGH! And my grades were disgusting!!!

5

Reason # 4 - Narrow, Little World

During medical school and residency, I felt squeezed into a narrow, little world. The medical school I attended generously provided "offices" for students, right there on the grounds. We could go from classroom to lab to library, and those offices were right there, on the way, waiting for us. We could cram in a few minutes or a few hours of studying any time, day or night.

Please don't misunderstand me. Providing those offices truly *was* a generous gesture by the school, and I think all my classmates and I appreciated having them. For, you see, we wanted to pass. We wanted to learn our course work, graduate from medical school, and become doctors. Having a handy cubicle for studying was a benefit. Plus, four students were assigned to each office, and there was a whole hallway full of offices, so we had help conveniently available almost all the time.

But we were a little bit like animals in a zoo, always in one cage or another, except when we went home at night.

Now, I know you're thinking, "Sure, maybe it was a confining world while you were learning and training, but eventually you escaped. Eventually, you became a doctor and got out of the cages. Right?"[13]

Okay, let's talk about that next.

6

Reason # 5 - The Buck Stops Here

I don't know how realistic I'm being now, but my perception was that, as a doctor, I would have to be seeing patients, reading medical journals, or attending CME courses (CME = continuing medical education) all the time. I would still be squeezing myself into a narrow, little world.

I had to find a way to always be ready for anything because whatever went wrong, it would be my fault. I couldn't pass the buck to anyone else. Whatever the "buck" is, I would be stuck with it.

I confess that my perception here may not be realistic because I didn't really like or enjoy the medical world. Therefore, I never felt adequately prepared. I had the sense that I didn't dare waste a minute doing anything not medical because…

Well, let's make a comparison with some other professions.

A waiter is daydreaming about his girlfriend and delivers the wrong order. His customer may yell at him, but he can simply go get the right order, solving the problem.

A teacher missed a day in teacher school and failed to learn an important fact. She provides faulty information to her class. That's bad, but chances are good that another teacher further on in her students' education process will correct the error, solving the problem.

A young man gets promoted to CEO because he's related to the company's owner. He doesn't have a clue what he's doing, and he runs the business into the ground. Chances are, that business is kaput. But look on the bright side - nobody died.

But if a doctor's expertise is faulty, a patient may suffer or die. That fact haunted me. I couldn't imagine being a doctor and not living in a narrow, little world of CME for fear I would fail to have the one vital fact that could save a life.

I was pretty sure I could cope with life as a doctor 40 or 50 hours per week. But in my view, the medical world was 24 hours a day, 365 days a year. It felt like a dark, endless tunnel.

And I'm claustrophobic!

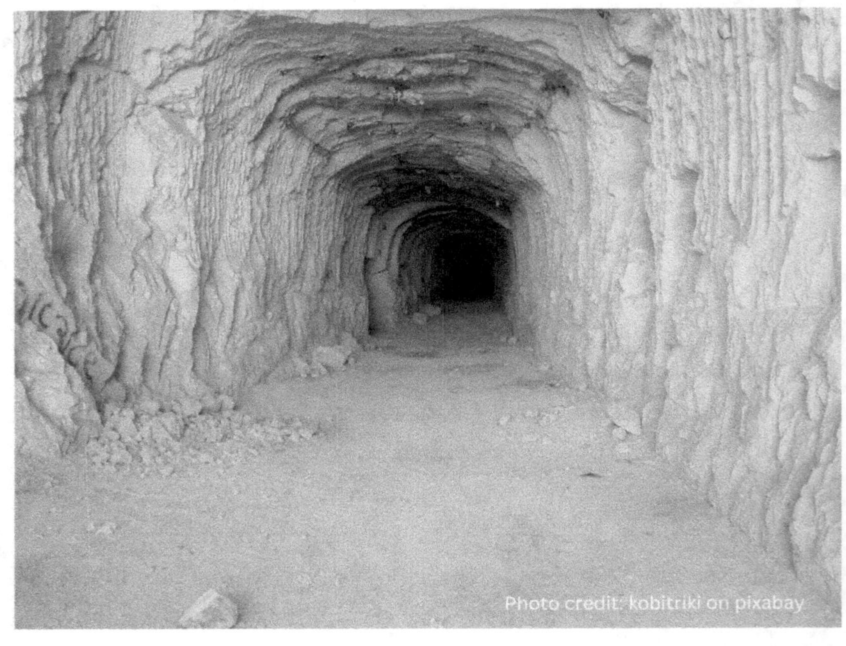
Photo credit: kobitriki on pixabay

7

Reason # 6 - Hopeless Cases

When I was a child, I lived in a park. My brothers and I ran wild - exploring, swinging, sliding, swimming, biking, playing tennis, etc. It was a magnificent childhood, and I used to think it was like living in Never Never Land. Except, unlike Peter Pan, our parents lived with us.

Of course, I wasn't ignorant of the fact that bad and sad situations existed in the world. It was just that such situations had little impact on my life. I was used to happy endings.

But the world of medicine is jam-packed with miserable, sorrowful endings. I still remember two examples from those early days.

The first was a little girl with a congenital heart defect. When I met her, she was in ICU and, if I remember right, she had just had surgery. She seemed to be doing well the first day. But she died the next day. She was a beautiful, gentle child, and I was horrified. My world went cattywampus. Babies were supposed to live, not die.

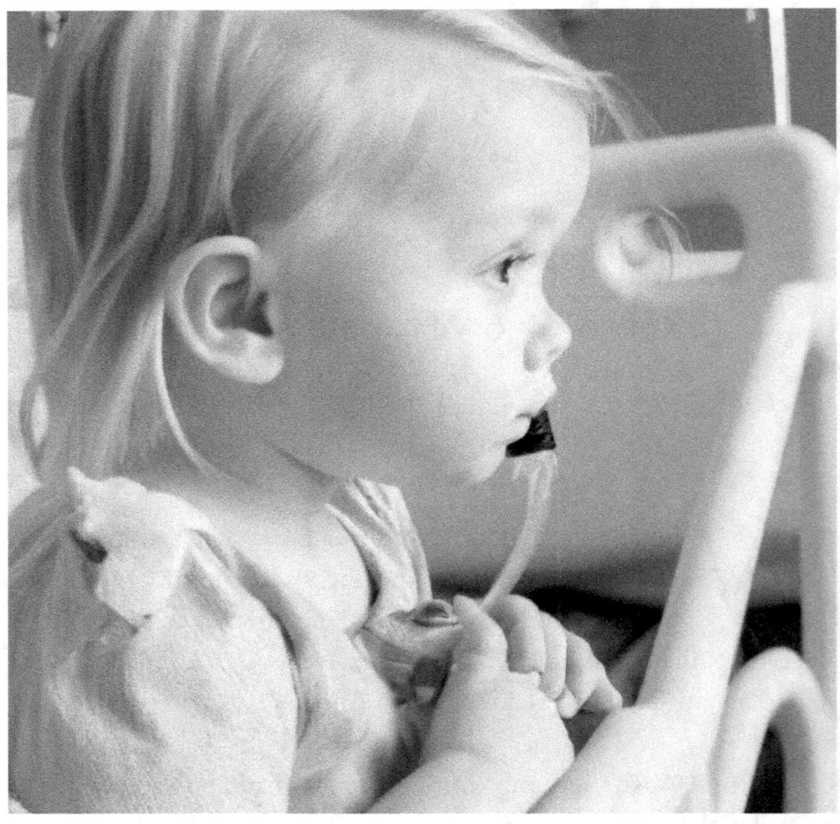

The other case was a woman in her 40's or 50's. She came to the hospital with asthma. First, she was in a private room, but her breathing deteriorated, and she was moved to the ICU. The first week, she grew sicker, then seemed to stabilize. The second week, she slowly, slowly began to improve. Finally, it looked like she was going to be strong enough to move out of ICU. Instead, she died suddenly. Again, my nicely-organized, Pollyannaish world staggered.

Okay, let's face it. Every patient is going to die. Maybe not right now, but we all die. And some will die under your care. Others may be crippled, require kidney dialysis or an amputation, suffer from unremitting pain or dementia, battle vicious cancers, etc. The medical world can be sad and ugly. God bless the doctors, nurses, and therapists who live in that world and battle the dragons, day in and day out. And if you choose to be one, kudos to you too.

8

Reason # 7 - A Personal Sorrow

I was in medical school in January, 1973, when the Supreme Court decreed that the murder of pre-born babies should be allowed in every state of the United States. It was one of the blackest days in the history of the nation I love.

There were many nights after that ruling when I could not sleep. Of course, I was deeply disturbed for my country. Billy Graham's wife, Ruth, once said that if God doesn't judge America, He will have to apologize to Sodom and Gomorrah. And I knew with all my heart that my beloved country would have to pay for the brutal destruction of its most helpless citizens.

However, most nights, it was not concern for my country that disturbed my sleep. It was torturous images of babies being torn apart. It was grievous dismay that a mother - any mother - could not only want, but demand the right, to kill her own child. How could Americans go on living with the knowledge that such barbarity was not only occurring, but occurring legally all around us?

Eventually, I found a way to cope with these sleep-slaughtering images. I truly believe that those precious little souls go from the "butcher block" straight into the arms of the Lord. It isn't what God wants. He ordains life, not death. But, as I reasoned at the time, a mother who was willing to spill the blood of her own child probably would not choose to raise her children in a godly home. Perhaps, many little ones ended up in Heaven who would not have made it otherwise.

With that conclusion, I regained my ability to sleep at night. I did not, however, lose a prevailing sense of grief and doom.

That's not the end of this story. During my final year in medical school, everyone in my class had to vote for the pledge we would take at our graduation ceremony. I still hear people referring to doctors taking the Hippocratic Oath as if it is a universal event in every medical school. But this was way back in 1975, and my class voted to take the "Declaration of Geneva," rather than the "Oath of Hippocrates."

Why did the great powers-that-be even put this choice before my class? Nobody ever told me, but it was probably because of this line from the "Oath of Hippocrates": "…and especially I will not aid a woman to procure abortion."

I didn't lead a protest march in favor of the Hippocratic Oath. And I didn't even think too much about it at the time. But now I can't help wondering if January 22, 1973, marked the beginning of a momentous decline in the ethics of a nation's doctors, as well as its citizens. Was medicine really the noble profession I had always believed it to be?

9

Reason # 8 - Money

We might as well talk about money. If I haven't scared you off yet, try this on for size. The average total cost for four years of medical school is $218,792! (The average yearly cost is $57,574.) This number includes tuition, fees, and health insurance. You still have to pay for food, lodging, transportation, etc. Expensive!

These numbers are from the website Education Data Initiative.[1] See "Resources" at the end of the book for the link if you would like to check the cost at a specific medical school.

Of course, the next question is how much will you make once you finish medical school and residency and are established in your practice. Here are some averages:

Average Doctor Annual Compensation by Specialty

Here are the top medical specialties, ranked by average income:

22

1. Plastic Surgery: $619,000
2. Orthopedics: $573,000
3. Cardiology: $507,000
4. Urology: $506,000
5. Gastroenterology: $501,000
6. Otolaryngology: $485,000
7. Radiology: $483,000
8. Oncology: $463,000
9. Anesthesiology: $448,000
10. Dermatology: $443,000
11. Surgery, General: $412,000
12. Critical Care: $406,000
13. Ophthalmology: $388,000
14. Pulmonary Medicine: $378,000
15. Emergency Medicine: $352,000
16. Pathology: $339,000
17. Ob/Gyn: $337,000
18. Neurology: $313,000
19. Nephrology: $312,000
20. Psychiatry: $309,000
21. Physical Medicine and Rehabilitation: $306,000
22. Allergy and Immunology: $282,000
23. Rheumatology: $281,000
24. Internal Medicine: $273,000
25. Diabetes and Endocrinology: $267,000
26. Infectious Diseases: $262,000
27. Family Medicine: $255,000
28. Pediatrics: $251,000
29. Public Health and Preventative Medicine: $249,000

Source: MedScape Physician Compensation Report, 2023

This information comes from the website Kaplan.[2] The link to the website is in the "Resources" section below.

.

Looking at these numbers, you may think you'll be making enough money as a doctor to easily pay off any student loans you accrue. Possibly. But don't forget that loans include interest charges. And you'll have to live. Plus, what if you go into private practice and have to set up an office?

Let's talk about that…

Here are some of the expenses to consider if you choose to set up your own practice:

Office space. You'll have to find a space with adequate facilities. If it's in a good location, like near the hospital, you can count on rent or purchase being expensive. Once you have it, you may want to make some changes. Does it need to be painted? Does it need new curtains or blinds or drapes? What about the plumbing - is it in good repair?

Office equipment and furniture. You, your nurse, your receptionist, your billing clerk, and perhaps others will need desks. Of course, you'll need a computer system, networked among all the offices. I don't even know how many chairs you might need; you'll need them for the lobby, the offices, and the examination rooms, at least. Even if you do most things electronically, you'll need filing cabinets. How about plants or paintings for the walls?

Office supplies. Now, this area is very important because it includes paper, envelopes, and stamps, so you can send out the bills! Maybe billing is handled electronically these days, but keep an eye on the system, whatever it is, and make sure it's glitch-free. You don't want your charges lost in cyberspace. Of course, this category includes staplers, tape, tissues, scissors, letterhead stationery, file folders and tabs, etc.

Medical equipment. Let's start with examination tables. You and your staff will need stethoscopes. Thermometers and blood pressure monitors are necessities. You may want a microscope and other lab equipment. You'd better have defibrillators. You need an accurate scale. You'll probably want to be able to do EKGs in your own office. A wheelchair or two might come in handy. Don't forget otoscopes and ophthalmoscopes. Let's leave it there. Depending on your specialty, you'll undoubtedly think of many more pieces of equipment you need.

Medical supplies. Here's a short list: exam gloves, syringes, sharps containers, alcohol swabs, cotton balls, bandages, paper and/or plastic cups, tongue depressors, paper towels, plastic wash basins, steri-strip skin closures, hydrogen peroxide, sterile gauze, specimen containers, bandage scissors, etc. You can see that stuff will add up.

Staff. You'll need a receptionist and a nurse, at the very least. And you'll have to have somebody to handle billing - whatever you do, make sure you have an honest, efficient person to manage the money. Expenses for your employees will include salaries, taxes and social security, health insurance, malpractice insurance for your nurse, and bonuses. It's a short list, but it's not cheap. And there may be other costs I haven't thought of.

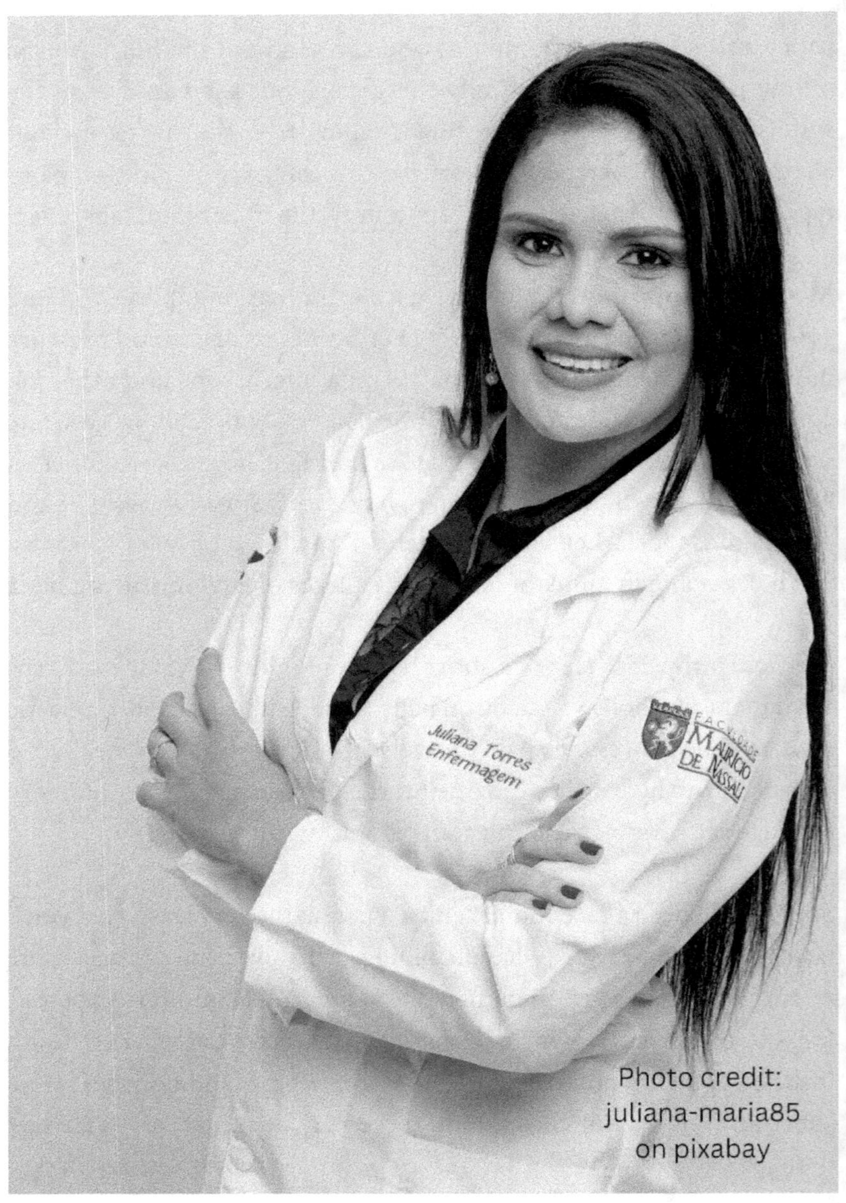

Malpractice insurance. Here are some averages from nerdwallet.com[3] for the cost to various specialists in various locations in the U.S. (A link to NerdWallet is in the Resources.)

Sample Annual Medical Malpractice Insurance Premiums, 2020

Obstetrics/Gynecology
   California (Los Angeles, Orange)$49,804
   Connecticut$134,054
   Florida (Miami-Dade)$205,380
   Illinois (Cook, Madison, St. Clair)$179,497
   New Jersey$90,749
   New York (Nassau, Suffolk)$174,552
   Pennsylvania (Philadelphia)$119,466

General surgery
   California (Los Angeles, Orange)$41,775
   Connecticut$90,577
   Florida (Miami-Dade)$205,380
   Illinois (Cook, Madison, St. Clair)$120,258
   New Jersey$60,810
   New York (Nassau, Suffolk)$154,056
   Pennsylvania (Philadelphia)$85,930

Internal medicine
   California (Los Angeles, Orange)$8,274
   Connecticut$18,878
   Florida (Miami-Dade)$51,345
   Illinois (Cook, Madison, St. Clair)$41,272
   New Jersey$15,900
   New York (Nassau, Suffolk)$33,852
   Pennsylvania (Philadelphia)$24,873

Nerd Wallet also adds the following information. Malpractice insurance generally covers attorney fees, court costs, arbitration fees, settlements, punitive and compensatory damages, and medical damages.

All things considered, you may decide to work for a hospital or join another doctor's practice. Even if you want a solo practice, you might make that a goal for after you've paid off your student debt. Another option for medical students is to join the military. If you do, much of the cost of your medical school education will be paid for you. However, you will then be required to serve in the military branch you joined, so this choice is not the best one unless you truly desire to spend some years serving in the military.

10

Reason # 9 - Emotional Toll

I'm sure you recognize there's an emotional toll associated with being a doctor. Physicians are exposed to a wide range of emotions every day, from the joy of helping a patient recover to the heartbreak of delivering a devastating diagnosis or witnessing a patient's suffering. This constant emotional roller coaster can take a toll on the doctor's mental and emotional well-being.

It's not uncommon for doctors to form strong connections with their patients. Then when patients face serious illness or even death, their caregivers may have deep feelings of helplessness and grief. The weight of responsibility in making critical decisions, coupled with the need to maintain composure in front of patients and their families, adds another layer of emotional stress. This emotional strain can lead to compassion fatigue, where healthcare providers become emotionally drained and may struggle to provide the same level of care over time. Additionally, the fear of making a mistake or missing a diagnosis can create anxiety and stress that impacts a doctor's overall mental health.

Imagine doctors as tightrope walkers, navigating a high wire stretched between realms of hope and despair. At one moment, they witness the jubilation of a patient's recovery, a feeling akin to successfully crossing the tightrope, arms raised in triumph. Another moment, the rope seems impossibly thin, as they deliver painful news. Tears stream down the face of the patient or a family member, and the doctor's balance falters. This delicate dance between joy and sorrow, life and death, defines the emotional tightrope doctors cross every day.

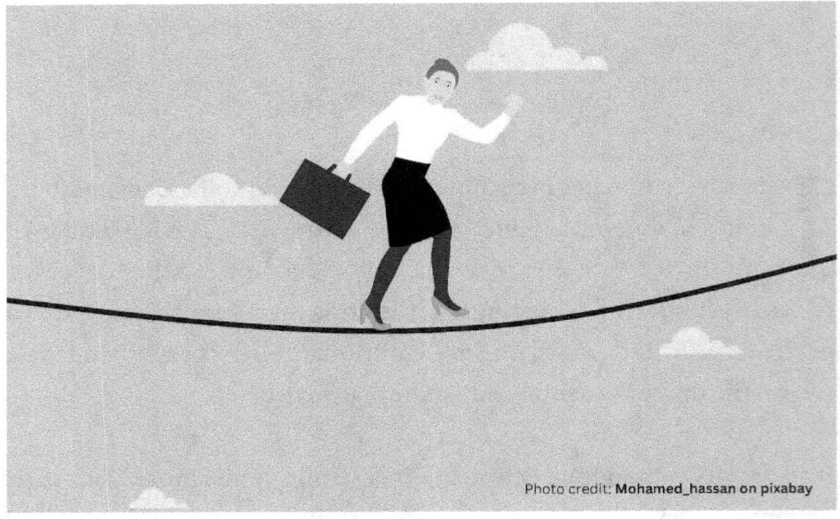

Photo credit: **Mohamed_hassan on pixabay**

As a doctor, it will be crucial for you to recognize and address the emotional toll on you for your own well-being, as well as for the quality of patient care you provide. When the time comes, consider using counseling services, peer support groups, or stress management classes. It will be your responsibility to prioritize self-care and seek support when you need it.

11

Reason # 10 - Physical Toll

The physical toll on doctors is a stark reality of the medical profession. Once you are in practice, you may find that modern doctors have found ways to reduce the constant bombardment of demands on their time. However, you still have to survive medical school and a residency. During those years, you will put in long hours every week. This drain on your time and energy can lead to exhaustion and burnout, as you will often be working late into the night and through weekends and holidays. The relentless schedule can disrupt sleep patterns and reduce your rest, which is so necessary for physical health. Also, your choice of a specialty may limit your ability to have free time - that's something to check out before you choose a specialty.

The demands of patient care can also take a physical toll. Some doctors must stand for extended periods during surgeries or rounds, leading to musculoskeletal issues such as back pain and joint problems. For example, orthopedic surgeons and anesthesiologists often experience physical strain due to the prolonged periods they spend on their feet. Additionally, the mental stress of making critical decisions and

31

managing complex medical cases can contribute to conditions like high blood pressure and heart disease.

Exposure to infectious diseases is another physical risk doctors face, particularly during outbreaks or pandemics. For instance, during the COVID-19 pandemic, healthcare workers were at heightened risk of contracting the virus due to their close proximity to infected patients. This not only puts their own health in jeopardy but also poses a risk to their families and communities.

Furthermore, the emotional toll on doctors can manifest physically as well. Stress and emotional exhaustion can contribute to symptoms like fatigue, headaches, and gastrointestinal problems. Keep it at the forefront of your mind that you must recognize and address the physical toll of your profession. It will be another of your responsibilities to institute self-care, to have regular health check-ups, and to seek support when you need it.

12

Reason # 11 - Commitment to Confidentiality

During a psychiatric rotation when I was in medical school, I came across a woman I knew from my hometown. I had access to her medical record and to sessions with her psychiatrist. To this day no one knows that I ever saw her in that psychiatric hospital. In fact, until now, no one even knows that I saw someone I knew in that situation.

Unless you can keep a secret - and that includes keeping secret that you have a secret - you don't belong in the medical profession. Some people, it seems, have a hard time not saying whatever comes to mind. And some of them can't help blabbing to a family member for the patient's "own good." Unauthorized sharing of medical information just isn't allowed, either ethically or legally.

But you're probably not the biggest problem. You're going to have a staff. How are you going to make sure your staff keep their mouths shut? I don't know the answer to that question, but it's something you'll need to figure out. Confidentiality in your office and hospital rotations must be a vault. Keep it locked and make sure nobody can get in unless they have your personal permission.

13

Reason # 12 - Family Sacrifices

I have an idea you can figure this one out without my help, but I'll make a couple of comments because this issue is so important.

First, exhaustion. Especially during medical school and residency, you will probably be exhausted all the time. Perhaps that is something you and your family should talk about ahead of time. Hopefully, just the fact that they've been forewarned will ward off some of their resentment and hard feelings if you fall asleep in the middle of dinner.

Second, priorities. You and your family may have different ideas about what your priorities should be. When your patients win out over your family for the 935th time, your spouse may begin to get a little miffed. And we all know that children spell love T-I-M-E. (So do spouses, by the way.) Anyway, I hope you will always find time to enjoy your family because they really do deserve to be your first priority.

Third, emotions. A doctor's job can have at least two unhealthy effects at home. What If you've been running late all day, your nurse was out sick, and your favorite patient suddenly presented with chest pain? You may be tempted to turn into a volcano at home, exploding at the least little thing your spouse or child does that irritates you. Or if you've been under a strain for days upon weeks or even months, you may not have any emotions left, at all. You just want to get in the bed and curl up in the fetal position.

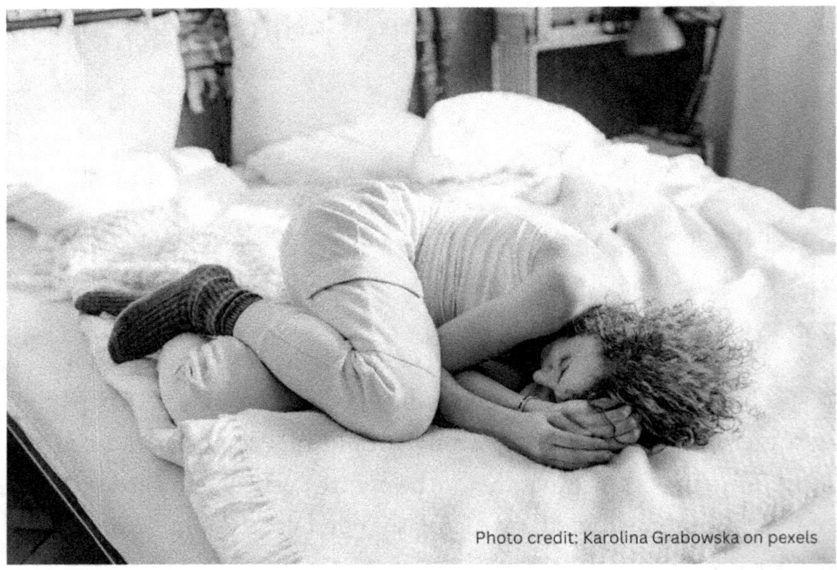

Photo credit: Karolina Grabowska on pexels

My opinion, for what it's worth, is that those are some issues you and your spouse should discuss before you start medical school - maybe come up with some solutions before you have the problems. Or if you're planning to get married after you're already in medical school or residency, warn your potential mate what he or she is getting into beforehand. Then you can prepare yourselves for the onslaught before you're in the middle of it. Or delay the wedding.

14

Reason # 13 - Regulations

Government regulations are an administrative burden on doctors. Plus, they can be expensive and eat into the doctor's clinical time. Of course, you already know that, and I don't have a lot of experience in this area. Anyway, it's a huge topic and you will be able to find all the information you need (and more) when the time comes. Just be aware that you'll have to deal with a mountain of regulations.

What I want to talk about in this section is the shocking, disgraceful behavior of the medical establishment during the COVID-19 pandemic. If you listen only to fake news, you may not be aware that effective treatments were available that would have reversed the disease in most patients. However, the government was putting pressure on doctors and nurses to employ treatments that either damaged or did not help patients. Honorable, courageous physicians who were providing genuine relief for their COVID-19 patients were ridiculed, and some lost hospital privileges.

As I understand it, the government paid hospitals for the care of COVID-

19 patients and paid extra when patients were put on ventilators. I don't know about any other part of the country, but around here, we despaired if someone we loved was put on a ventilator. It felt like a death sentence. On the other hand, simple, relatively inexpensive treatments like Hydroxychloroquine tabs, Ivermectin tabs, and Budesonide delivered through a nebulizer were reported to be effective in almost all cases where they were used.

Personally, I took Vitamin D, Vitamin C, Zinc, and Quercetin prophylactically, and I never got the virus. But I didn't hear from the fake news media or any other ordinary channels that these products could help keep me safe. Instead, I had to hear it from news sources who were being called liars by the government and its agents.

So, I want to ask you this question. What would you do if an authority figure told you that you must withhold an effective medication from a seriously ill patient and instead administer a medication that could do harm if it had any effect at all?

That situation could arise again. And just so you know, if you choose to obey the government at the expense of your patient, you'll be breaking your pledge, whether you took the "Declaration of Geneva" or the "Oath of Hippocrates."

I'll cite some websites in the Resources in case you're interested in this topic.[4]

15

Conclusion

Now to finish my story...

After medical school, I worked a couple of years in a government clinic - 40 hours a week, and home at night with no call, no hospital duties. That was a dream! But then I felt obliged to start a residency. I signed up for a year, and I don't believe one of those 365 days passed without my fantasizing a way to get out of it early.

What if my apartment building burned down, and everyone thought I was dead?

What if I packed up and moved away, letting everyone wonder where I went?

What if the President of the United States sent for me because he had an urgent assignment for me?

Obviously, those were a pack of ridiculous, unrealistic fantasies. And yet, I remember that when I was down to the last two weeks, I was still trying to think of a valid way to keep from doing those last two weeks. I can't begin to tell you how miserable I was and how much I hated the practice of medicine. I hated it more than cockroaches!

Well, the 365th day finally arrived. I walked out of the hospital and never looked back. A few years later, I quit renewing my medical license because I didn't ever want to be tempted to go back, just because I was hungry or homeless or facing some other minor crisis.

And that's my story.

The Only Good Reason

Now let me tell you the only good reason - in my opinion - anyone should become a practicing physician...

But first, did you notice I said PRACTICING physician? You see, there are other options after medical school. For example, medical research, hospital administration, medical technology, education, writing, and others. Some medical school graduates earn another degree - law or business, for example.

So, I'm not talking about those cases. I'm talking about a clinical physician who cares for patients as his/her main occupation. My opinion is that the only good reason to become one of those is the *love of medicine*. When I say the "love of medicine," I'm talking about human anatomy and physiology, the mystery of pathology, and the solutions: pharmaceuticals, surgery, and/or other therapies. Practicing physicians need to LOVE the whole package.

There are a lot of reasons people become doctors. But let's say I had to choose a doctor, and my choice was among a) someone who went into medicine to earn a lot of money, b) someone who has a world-class bedside manner, and c) someone who went into medicine for the pure love of medicine. I would choose the one who loves medicine every time.

If you have a heart for people and a love of medicine, I hope you'll ignore my 13 reasons and become a doctor. You'll be a good one!

As a Favor...

...if you enjoyed this book or if it helped you in any way, would you please write a smashing-good review about it on amazon.com? I would be most grateful.

16

Resources

[1] Hanson, M. (2023, July 12). Average cost of medical school [2023]: yearly + total costs. Education Data Initiative. https://educationdata.org/average-cost-of-medical-school

[2] Admin. (2023, June 14). Average doctor salaries by specialty. https://www.kaptest.com/study/mcat/doctor-salaries-by-specialty/

[3] Orem, T. (2023). How much is malpractice insurance? NerdWallet. https://www.nerdwallet.com/article/small-business/how-much-is-malpractice-insurance

[4] The COVID scandal

Aflds. (n.d.). Home | America's Frontline Doctors. America's Frontline Doctors. https://americasfrontlinedoctors.org/

Followers, O. T. M. 4. (n.d.). Covid chaos: conspiracy or reality? (Part 1) – Twila Brase and Marjorie Holsten [Video]. Rumble. https://rumble.com/vsjizc-covid-chaos-conspiracy-or-reality-part-1-twila-brase-

and-marjorie-holsten.html

Followers, O. T. M. 4. (n.d.-b). Covid chaos: conspiracy or reality? (Part 1) – Twila Brase and Marjorie Holsten [Video]. Rumble. https://rumble.com/vsjizc-covid-chaos-conspiracy-or-reality-part-1-twila-brase-and-marjorie-holsten.html

Followers, O. T. M. 4. (n.d.-c). Covid chaos: conspiracy or reality? (Part 2) – Twila Brase and Marjorie Holsten [Video]. Rumble. https://rumble.com/vsyyf7-covid-chaos-conspiracy-or-reality-part-2-twila-brase-and-marjorie-holsten.html

Olive Tree Ministries. (2023, July 1). Breaking the oath - Olive tree ministries. https://olivetreeviews.org/radio-archives/breaking-the-oath/

Our Amazing Grace: Tragedy behind the hospital that killed Grace. (n.d.). https://ouramazinggrace.net/Tragedy-hospital